ENDORSEMENTS

"Jill's passion for uncovering each layer of a patient's overall health is not only admirable, but she's also highly effective. She truly cares about identifying root cause issues to improve her patient's (and family's) quality of life. She's a solutions-oriented doctor."

Dr. Keith Thornton, Founder, and Chairman,
Airway Management
Charles Collins, CEO, Airway Management

"Dr. Jill Ombrello is not only a great friend of many years but a respected professional colleague as well. Many years ago, I was giving a seminar on early orthodontics in California, and an attending dentist raised her hand and stated that her father was a dentist and had straightened her teeth as a youngster with the appliance we were lecturing on. I invited her to come up and tell the audience about her experience. The manner in which she explained this to the audience convinced me that she had an unbelievable talent as a public speaker. Our friendship began on that day. Since that time, Dr. Ombrello has given hundreds of lectures educating the profession regarding her holistic approach to sleep problems and orthodontic treatment procedures for both children and adults.

Having known Dr. Ombrello's unique natural approach to all aspects of dental care and her relentless pursuit of the causes of various problems, I have realized that she has not only educated fellow professionals but has imparted her knowledge and conservative dental philosophy to improve the future health and well-being for many adults but also for their children as well. Her relentless pursuit of not only the causes of dental and abnormal sleep health issues but of the most conservative methods of her treatment of these same issues is to be commended.

Having known Dr. Ombrello for so many years has been a privilege and has given me a unique understanding of what a dental professional should be regarding their unselfish service to their patients. A read of this book will give you the same understanding of Jill's dental philosophy as I have had the privilege of experiencing. Thank you, Dr. Ombrello."

Dr. Earl Bergersen, Innovator for Interceptive Orthodontics and Inventor of Orthotain/ Healthy Start

"Dr. Jill Ombrello is a talented provider and lecturer that keeps the audience on their toes and challenges them to get out of their comfort zone. Her passion and her no-nonsense unapologetic approach are refreshing and fun. Always proud and happy to share the stage with her whenever the opportunity arises."

David Galler, AACA - The American Academy of Clear Aligners

"This is an endorsement for one of the best dentists I have ever known. The endorsement is actually not for Dr. Jill Ombrello the dentist, but for Jill Ombrello the person. One of Jill's best characteristics is that she always tries to do "the right thing." One of my best memories of the character of Jill is running a lap around the playground by holding the hand of her blind classmate. Jill is the true definition of a kind person."

Dr. Michael Rosellini

Moms in the Trenches

Moms in the Trenches

How Moms Can Unpack the Root Cause,
Advocate for their Children's Health,
and Join the Other Side

DR. JILL OMBRELLO, MOM

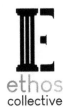

ethos
collective

Moms in the Trenches ©2023 Dr. Jill Ombrello, MOM.

Published by Ethos Collective™
PO Box 43, Powell, OH 43065
www.ethoscollective.vip

Library of Congress Cataloging: 2023902717
Softcover: 978-1-63680-128-5
Hardcover: 978-1-63680-129-2
E-book: 978-1-63680-130-8
Available in hardcover, softcover, e-book, and audiobook.

DEDICATION

To Franny, Vinny, Gino, and Eloise, the four most beautiful people who made me a mom. Thank you for making me question, learn and discover constantly. You are my why. And to Jimbo, my everything. Thank you for this beautiful life and for showing me what true love feels like. And to all the moms who join me in the trenches to make each child the best and healthiest version of themselves.

CONTENTS

FOREWORD

After hearing Dr. Jill Ombrello speak for 5 minutes, I knew I liked her. What she said got my attention, but how she said it captured my heart. Her words contained data and stories, but her tone oozed with conviction and passion.

I knew I met someone special.

Here was an expert with decades of experience but also a mom who was literally in the trenches, fighting the battle of protecting her kids. Her wisdom contained wounds and battle scars. The more she shared I could tell she was winning the war.

After hearing her story, I realized the source of her strength. She had walked this way before in her own health journey. As a young adult, she had to trust her gut when medical professionals weren't listening to her pleas for help.

It wasn't a waste. She converted her pain into a promise. If she became a healthcare provider, she would listen to her patients, not just prescribe medicine. She committed to exploring the root causes behind the presenting problem.

Today, Dr. Jill Ombrello and her team at Central Dentist offer diverse services, including early intervention orthodontics, periodontal therapies, airway evaluation, ceramic biocompatible implants, ozone treatments, TMD therapy, and cosmetic smile makeovers.

Her practice helps patients:

- Understand the path to sustainable health so they can enjoy lasting wellness.

- Learn healthcare options so they can make the best-informed choices.

- Advocate for health so her patients experience a better future.

The best news is that you don't have to travel to Texas for a solution. *Moms In the Trenches* will give you and your family the tools you need to advocate for your children's health.

Hope and healing is possible. Get ready to join the other side.

Dr. Kary Oberbrunner, Wall Street Journal and USA Today bestselling author of 13 books, CEO Igniting Souls

A NOTE TO YOU— THE READER

Dearest reader,

I've never shared the details of this story with anyone outside my most inner circle who went through it with me. I decided it was time. It's time to be transparent, heal, and truly explain my ferocious passion to empower others to understand how to become the best version of themselves.

Thank you for going on this journey with me.

Jill

INTRODUCTION:
I SHOULD BE HAPPY

I don't want to live one more day like this. Darkness overtook my usually extroverted glass-half-full personality. Constantly sick, my energy sapped; I couldn't walk up a set of stairs.

Dental school was my dream, but my friends had to carry my backpack, and my brother dropped out of law school in New York to take care of me in Houston. Mom made frozen meals so I had something healthy to eat, and my lovely independent life turned to complete dependency.

I should've been happy. What was my problem? Where did things go wrong?

Borderline suicidal and terrified, I decided this would not be my reality. That decision was the first step. The second step was to redefine my story.

NOBODY BELIEVED ME

My symptoms first surfaced in 2000. I was a high-achieving freshman in college playing Division One field hockey, making good grades, and running half marathons, until the stroke. I was driving my car and lost vision in my eye, and I rear-ended the vehicle in front of me. Everyone walked away ok, but that moment changed everything for me.

I saw every specialist from St. Louis to Dallas. They asked all kinds of demeaning and condescending questions. Was the incident alcohol or drug-related? Did I have multiple sclerosis? Each question made me feel like I had done this to myself.

Eventually, I was honest with them. "I've been having these spells for seven years. I thought it was normal to get dizzy and fall over. The loss of eyesight in my right eye was temporary every time. So, I figured I was okay, right?"

Addressing my strokes (or mini-strokes known as trans ischemic attacks in the medical world) opened my eyes, forcing me to realize my high-achieving glass-half-full attitude had convinced me to live with symptoms rather than discover what caused them.

During the diagnostic process, a doctor told me I needed open heart surgery. With no other options, this was my new reality. I was a great compensator. I learned exactly what to do when I got dizzy and lost my vision. A funny comment distracted those that noticed. I had this under control until I didn't.

I felt extreme support from my incredible parents and boyfriend—now my husband. To say I was a disagreeable or uncooperative patient would be an understatement. I thought I could will myself better or just push through until I recovered.

The doctor performed the surgery, but the procedure didn't go well. For the next year, I felt worse than before I had heart surgery.

With swollen legs, red face, and always out of breath, I became emotional and developed allergies to products I had used for years. One over-the-counter nasal spray caused burns inside my nose that took weeks to heal. How could my body change so much from a procedure that was supposed to help me?

The worst part of the entire ordeal—my doctor told me the symptoms existed only in my mind. He called me weak and said I needed to work harder to feel better. The variety of diagnoses and accusations was overwhelming—Multiple Sclerosis, addictions, neurological abnormalities. Nobody believed me, so I began not to believe or trust myself. I couldn't figure out why my boyfriend didn't break up with me and find someone who could have fun, be healthy, and have more energy. I felt lower than low most days.

Doctors are human, and my doctor messed up. I had every right to hold on to the anger because he messed up on me, but I needed to move on. So I asked myself: *what am I going to do to get better?*

An unstoppable and undeniable survival instinct surfaced. I knew I had to find a different way to look at my situation and started to trust my gut. My health experience wasn't typical. I needed to educate myself on other options. Desperation drove me.

With the unwavering support from my family and Jim, I decided to fight—against the world. I may have been the shell of a past me at the moment, but I am determined to find the healthy, happy, and full of gratitude version of me I knew existed.

YOU HAVE TO HELP ME

My boyfriend, a soon-to-be husband, worked in physical therapy at The University of Texas MD Anderson Cancer Center in the bone marrow transplant department.

During my lowest days, one of his patients was a cardiologist. My situation came up in his patient's twice-daily rehab routine. While I have no doubt my husband helped this man recover from cancer, I believe God placed this person in our lives at just the right moment. Of all the patients Jim could have treated, God placed someone with insight and information that allowed Jim to take the following steps that ultimately saved my life.

This cardiologist unofficially examined a copy of my transesophageal echocardiogram, a heart ultrasound. He took one look and told my husband he saw something very wrong.

I was fed up with feeling sick and being completely dysfunctional, so I took his advice and walked from the dental school to St. Luke's Hospital next door. I found the directory screen, and divine intervention led me to Dr. Charles Fraser, the chief of pediatric cardiothoracic surgery.

My dental school scrubs took me past the front desk, and I waved at the receptionist as I continued through a crowd of waiting patients and directly into the chief of cardiothoracic surgery's office. He was a badass, top-dog doctor. Who was I to just walk in? (I found out later that my mom's dearest long-term teacher friend, Kathy Miller, made a call to Dr. Fraser on my behalf, letting him know the details of my situation and to be expecting me. I still get goosebumps of gratitude when I reflect on how friends of the family know friends and call in favors that ultimately saved my life. The world is a beautiful place full of people eager to help each other.)

I learned a lesson that day—one I reinforced to my kids: you have to ask for what you want. Ask for forgiveness rather than permission. No one will just hand anything to you. I never want my children to hesitate. I want them to walk through the crowd's room, knock down doors, and make their voices and concerns heard, even when they feel like no one is listening.

Dr. Fraser was hosting an international meeting with cardiovascular surgeons at the time. At one point, he stepped out of the meeting to get something from his office, and he found me sitting there. Unfazed by my presence, he asked, "How can I help you today?"

"You have to help me." And with tears, I told him my story. I felt like I spoke forever though it was probably only about five minutes. I gave him as much info as I could in the short time he didn't really have, and I didn't deserve it. I begged him to view my post-surgery TEE, and he decided it was compelling enough to show it to the other doctors in his meeting during their fifteen-minute break.

Over one hundred international cardiothoracic surgeons viewed my TEE. What were the odds of such a prestigious group meeting on this day in this building?

Dr. Fraser later said the entire audience gasped when he showed the image of my heart. They couldn't believe what they saw or that I was still alive.

Those doctors diagnosed me with patent foramen ovale (PFO). Essentially, a tube in one chamber of the heart brings blood up from the bottom of your body. Your heart processes it and pumps it all around the four chambers. It takes oxygenated blood through a different artery to your entire body. Oxygen is the key ingredient here. You can go weeks without food, days without water but only minutes without oxygen.

When you're a baby, you have a hole in between the two chambers of your heart because your mother oxygenated your blood for you. When you're born, the pressure in your heart changes so that a little flap closes the hole. Now you oxygenate your blood on your own.

In 20% of the population, that flap never closes. Only 5% have symptoms, so a PFO diagnosis is rare. Doctors must rule out everything else before blaming PFO for the symptoms.

When my first doctor tied the hole closed, he also caught part of the tube that delivers the under-oxygenated blood as well.

Not one of those specialists could believe that the surgeon had sutured part of my inferior vena cava. They wanted to meet me, but Dr. Fraser said I wasn't stable, and he scheduled me for open heart surgery the next morning. I called my parents from Dr. Fraser's office and could hear the fright and relief in their voices as they said they would travel to Houston immediately. As a parent now, I can't even imagine how my parents felt at this moment, but I appreciated them coming to Houston immediately because I was scared.

I am overwhelmed with gratitude that Dr. Fraser prioritized and protected me in that moment. I was not mentally, emotionally, or physically ready to hear that gasp or answer their questions. After a fifteen-minute meeting, Dr. Fraser showed compassion, care, and love for me that no other doctor had ever shown.

I spent fourteen months before meeting Dr. Fraser in a state of fight or flight. I always tell my patients that we have parasympathetic and sympathetic systems. The parasympathetic system allows us to be calm and aids in rest and digestion. The sympathetic system prepares us for stress and strenuous activity. The constant vigilant system is what we call fight or flight syndrome.

Our bodies don't function well in that state for an extended period. It doesn't let us rest or detox properly and raises cortisol levels.

Extended sympathetic states come from compromised airways, incorrect nighttime breathing, bad posture, or poor nutrition. Shifting our bodies corrects and addresses those root causes and gets us back into a parasympathetic state. With the correct intervention, our bodies can adjust within approximately thirty days, though often, patients feel worse before they feel better. But as cortisol levels return to normal and the body begins to heal from the trauma it has been compensating for, the turnaround becomes amazing, and it's worth the month-long wait.

It is miraculous how quickly the body can heal when functioning correctly. I immediately felt better after my second open-heart surgery.

My philosophy of care focuses on healing, proper sleep, and oxygenated breathing too to restore proper body function. Many patients come into my office on their thirty-day appointment with happy tears, filled with gratitude. After those thirty days, their health improves, and they trust me as they begin to feel the positive results of treatment. Most feel regret and anger after suffering through life for so long, but even more, they express gratitude because they feel so much better. Grateful they identified and addressed the root cause of their symptoms, they begin to believe their body can continue to heal.

"Is this how everybody else feels?" "Why didn't someone tell me?" "Why didn't I do this sooner?" "Why doesn't everybody know this?"

We can see such positive benefits by introducing a simple solution that aligns the body with its proper function.

My patients, like me and maybe you, deal with the suffering and just try to do their best. They can't remember what feeling good feels like.

When my symptoms were diagnosed, and a treatment option was laid out for me, I felt like I could finally hope again, just like my patients.

UNDER THE KNIFE

Before my second heart surgery, fear consumed me. *Do I understand what this doctor plans to do? Can I trust this surgeon? After all, I trusted the last one. Will I ever be better? What will happen to my dreams? Will I be worse the second time I wake up?*

My first surgery was done by one of the best cardiologists in the country. However, he neglected to give me options or empower me to make the best decision for me. Instead, he left me feeling scared and backed into a corner. My experience taught me to always advocate for myself and my family.

I CAN BREATHE

I woke from that second seven-hour surgery feeling very different from the first. One of the first things I did was take a huge, deep breath.

"I can breathe!" I said just before I started to cry. I began to remember how what a healthy body felt like.

My first surgery left me unable to breathe correctly, and the doctor told me shortness of breath, a swollen face, and an enlarged liver would define my future; I should learn to deal with them.

So, even though I had just faced horrendous open-heart surgery, including a broken sternum and ribs, I was amazed that I could breathe. My body could finally function the way it was supposed to. I knew recovery would be an uphill battle, but filling my lungs gave me confidence that better days were waiting.

Excited and motivated by my ability to breathe, improved health, and clear head, I wanted to prove to myself and my doctors that I could return to the life I loved.

Six months after my second surgery, I ran the Houston half marathon with my best friend Niki. Dr. Fraser greeted me with a poster cheering me on. I'm sure thousands of patients have similar stories about him. But at the time, he made me feel I was his most important patient.

I later learned that on the day Dr. Fraser performed my surgery, he was supposed to be boarding an airplane for his first vacation in five years. Instead, he sent his family to the ski resort and gave me my life back. I can only imagine the flack he took for putting work before family. I catch a glimpse now and then when I'm late for dinner or a soccer game because I'm finishing up treatment or answering a patient's questions. I strive to follow his example of what a doctor is supposed to be. He serves wholeheartedly and puts the patient's interests first. I still send him a Christmas card every year.

When I crossed that half-marathon finish line, I knew I was back. I was still an athlete who could work hard and achieve new goals.

Before becoming a mom, I stepped into the trenches and fought for myself.

IN THE TRENCHES

For a long time after my surgeries, I harbored an unhealthy amount of anger and resentment toward the first doctor. Initially, his discovery of my issue made me grateful. But after I realized I'd lost at least a year of my life, I grew angry and resentful. My problem could have been resolved with pharmaceutics. But he never offered options other than surgery.

Anger, heartbreak, and blame drove me for a time; however, little by little, I learned to thank him for teaching me a lesson. I will never allow my perceived authority as an expert in the dental field to decide for someone else. I have my own bias. Still, I am determined always to present every single option. Even if some options mean referrals, I want my patients to have all the information necessary to figure out what works best for them.

That first surgeon's mistake has embedded in me the significance of the vows I shared with my husband. He promised to stick by me in sickness and health, but he proved it long before our marriage. My ordeal helped me understand a parent's love for their child. And now that I have children of my own, I know the physical pain and helplessness my parents felt while watching their child struggle. In the end, I also learned the value of true friendship. Training for a half marathon with a friend recovering from heart surgery requires a level of patience and love and few experiences. I was so blessed to have Niki run with me. She also supplied endless celebrity gossip and Beyonce songs to help quickly pass the time on our longer training runs. I feel unwavering gratitude for all the people in my life.

I saw that first doctor in a grocery store years later. When he noticed me, he became physically uncomfortable and sought a place to retreat. I can only imagine what he thought I would say. I felt a new level of self-satisfaction when I looked him in the eyes and said, "Thank you."

Full disclosure: This was our second meeting. Our first encounter involved many four-letter words I would hate for my mom and children to read in this book. But by the second time our paths crossed, I had healed physically and emotionally.

Doctors don't always need to introduce treatment options that aren't natural.

In my field, many patients face uncomfortable metal braces or unnecessary pharmaceutical solutions. Wouldn't it be better to figure out why the body is trying to compensate with mouth breathing, grinding teeth, and snoring? By addressing the root cause, our miraculous and magical bodies will do what they should.

My year of desperation pushes me to search relentlessly for the origin of my patient's symptoms. I eventually moved past the resentment that built for the first surgeon. The experience made me a better doctor and a better person. Despite the first surgeon's mistakes, I have become someone who fights alongside others and guides them through the trenches that I battled in for years.

PART ONE

PROBLEM

1

UNDERSTANDING THE BASICS

When my first daughter was three, she began having night terrors. Her shrieks in the middle of the night sent me running to her room, only to find her crying and upset but still asleep.

After countless nights of these horrific dreams, I began to worry, so I called her pediatrician. He told me it was normal. I didn't say anything, but I disagreed. Maybe these nightmares are common, but they are not normal.

It's time to stop accepting a problem or issue simply because there doesn't seem to be a solution. A sweet little three-year-old screaming in the middle of the night should not be considered commonplace. Someone should look for answers. I decided I would find other options to help my daughter.

My daughter's nightmares started driving my actions as a parent, and I fight an uphill battle daily to be an advocate for my children's health.

Every parent needs to advocate for their kids' health. We shouldn't settle for mediocre options. Instead, we should insist someone look for the *root* causes and empower ourselves to upend what's considered normal.

My daughter regularly suffered from oxygen desaturation events throughout the night because she was a mouth breather. A simple oral device took care of the problem. After she got enough oxygen at night, she enjoyed restful, restorative sleep free from night terrors and other symptoms.

As a society, we are drowning in chronic disease. Children suffer from headaches, snoring, asthma, prolonged bed wetting, difficulty focusing mentally, anxiety, and difficulty sleeping. Adults fare about as well. They endure cardiovascular disease, poor sleep, thyroid problems, and autoimmune disease. Of course, many factors can contribute to these problems, but medical practitioners rarely consider one factor.

Understanding our origins is important to grasp life's problems today. Travel back more than 10,000 years before the development of agriculture. Our ancestors lived in nature, hunting and gathering food. They never concerned themselves about access to uncontaminated water and clean ingredients. These hunter-gatherers ate meat, fruit, nuts, wild grains, and vegetables. Most of the food was difficult to chew, forcing humans to use their facial muscles to really break it down before swallowing.

The introduction of softer diet thousands of years later eliminated the need to exercise our jaws and began to change the shapes of our faces. We now see narrower jaws, which causes restricted airways. Smaller mandibles leave less room for teeth and force the tongue backward into the airway, especially during sleep.

As the other facial bones devolved, nasal passages shrank, too. While all the contributing factors can be overwhelming for a parent of a struggling child, our goal is to create an understanding of how the body is supposed to work so each parent can act as an advocate for their child and treat the root cause rather than the symptoms. Dr. Weston Price did years of research measuring this evolutionary change seen in humans in his book *Nutrition and Physical Degeneration.*[10]

FOOD AND WATER

Humans need food and water to survive. Yet, these essentials look different than when our grandparents built their families.

Everybody assumes their city delivers clean water, but you might be surprised at the bacteria in your city's water supply. Plus, many cities add fluoride, a neurotoxin. Three decades of solvent-filled water in Camp Lejune, lead in the water in Flint, Michigan, and a 2023 train derailment in Ohio emptying tankers full of toxic liquid into the environment prove we must advocate for clean water.

You can check public records online to see the status of your city's water supply. Information about what you put in your body will empower you to make healthy decisions.

Perhaps you think bottled water is the answer. Unfortunately, the plastic's BPA leaches into the contents and affects women's estrogen levels, thyroid, and, potentially, their fertility. Even those who understand the risks tend to think drinking one bottle won't hurt. But if you drink one every day, it absolutely will.

Water and soil quality in the twenty-first century is poor. Plus, food is commercially packaged in plastic that can break down and leak into your food. A recent study found that the average person eats five grams of microplastics weekly.[10] You may as well steam your credit card and eat it.

In addition, the University of Vienna suggests, "Ingested particles passing through the gastrointestinal tract lead to changes in the composition of the gut microbiome. These changes are linked to metabolic diseases like obesity, diabetes, and chronic liver disease. The particles can trigger local inflammation and immune response, and nano plastics, in particular, have been found to trigger chemical pathways involved in the formation of cancer."[10]

Most consumers don't understand the evolution of toxins introduced into our environment since the Industrial Revolution. Our grandparents' rules to live a healthy life do not apply to our children. When we add disturbed sleep patterns to the mix, we discover liver toxicity and a compromised ability to respond to our environment, setting us up for a lifetime of trying to compensate and eventual sickness.

BREATHING

Imagine having difficulty breathing while you sleep, so much so that your body jolts itself awake a few times every hour as your body gasps for air. Even if you don't know what woke you, your body will feel the effects: complete exhaustion, irritability, aggression, anxiety, difficulty concentrating, etc.

Many symptoms include migraines, ADD/ADHD, depression, allergies, chronic pain, and inflammation. This silent epidemic affects nine out of ten children. Often, physicians ignore the signs and symptoms, disregarding them as "a phase" or misdiagnosing them as a different disorder.

As a practitioner and as a mom, my philosophy is to evaluate the "whole person" and to collaborate with other like-minded healthcare providers to enhance our knowledge of the issues. We look for the root cause and provide all options, something I wish doctors had done for me with my heart surgery. Each day these kids go undiagnosed, their condition worsens, their potential for growth and development diminishes, and the window of time to treat them narrows.

ORAL REST POSTURE

Have you ever heard of Oral Rest Posture? When our oral and facial muscles are at rest, our tongue should be against the roof of the mouth, our lips should be sealed, and our jaws should be closed with only a few millimeters of space between the teeth. When this posture is disturbed, the tongue will often sit too far forward in your mouth. Many things can alter a good Oral Rest Posture, including chronic mouth breathing, allergies, enlarged tonsils or adenoids, and an untreated tongue tie. In addition, prolonged thumb, pacifier, or sippy cup use teaches the tongue to rest in the wrong position.

We can get caught in a vicious cycle without proper Oral Rest and Tongue Posture. Everything that forces us to mouth breathe can also be a symptom. Mouth breathing forces tonsils and adenoids to humidify and purify air instead of the nose, which has built-in filters called cilia. When the tonsils and adenoids have to do the work, they begin to swell.

Mouth breathing doesn't take care of germs either—germs that can more easily infect compromised and enlarged adenoids and tonsils. And the cycle completes itself because sleep-disordered breathing is more common in children with enlarged tonsils and adenoids. Compromised immunity, sore throats, and swollen tonsils make parents desperate to get off of this merry-go-round of antibiotics and sickness.

You would think a tonsillectomy is especially they are among the most frequently performed surgical procedures on children in the United States.[12] However, tonsils and adenoids are not like fingers. If you cut off a finger, your finger is gone forever. Tonsils and adenoids are tissue, so when a surgeon removes them, that lymphatic tissue lives on. The tissue can become inflamed again, and kids get right back on the merry-go-round.

Poor Oral Rest Posture can also lead to delayed speech, creating frustration and affecting their little personalities as they begin communicating their thoughts and ideas.

Various treatment options, including tonsillectomy and adenoidectomy (removal of tonsils and adenoids, removal of the back third of the tongue, and even implantable nerve stimulators like Inspire, which fire off during sleep) are scary treatment options for parents.

DOCTOR GOOGLE IS NOT THE BEST

Raise your hand if you've had a symptom, such as chest pain, headaches, rash, etc., and open Google to find the cause. Indeed someone on Instagram or TikTok has advice. And don't forget to plug in their code for a discount so they receive their kickback.

After all your "research," you decide you are either having a heart attack or contracting some flesh-eating bacteria.

An article from *Neuroscience News* states, "Many people turn to 'Dr. Google' to self-diagnose their health symptoms and seek medical advice, but online symptom checkers are only accurate about a third of the time, according to new Edith Cowan University (ECU) research published in the *Medical Journal of Australia* today."[1]

Another article from Cleveland Station WYKC states, "A 2013 study found that WebMD received more money from pharmaceutical and device companies than any other medical communication company. Therefore, they report on the companies they are receiving money from." [2] Big pharma is not our friend. The same study mentioned that WebMD listed the correct diagnosis first in only 34% of patient evaluations.

In this information age, everybody knows everything and has an opinion. Most speak with no credentials but plenty of offensive and divisive thoughts. Many moms have difficulty asking whether a vaccine or medicine is suitable for their children. They fear someone will chastise or shame them. But asking questions and empowering yourself is the right thing to do. If you feel shame for asking, you need a different medical professional or facility.

AMAZON IS NOT YOUR HEALTH PROVIDER

Yes, you can search Amazon for health advice, not only through their main shopping pages but as a clinic. Even though Amazon Care, Amazon's version of telehealth, ceased to exist in December 2022,[3] Amazon Pharmacy and Clinic continue to operate.

With Amazon Clinic, you don't need an appointment. You simply enter your symptoms, a clinician reviews them, and then you get treated. The result is a full list of products they could buy to solve their problem. I think this is an analysis by paralysis type of mentality that I see in so many moms and patients.

When kids have an issue, like thumb-sucking, Amazon has an answer. Within seconds you'll see a page with a host of products you can purchase to "solve" thumb sucking, or mouth breathing, or whatever it may be. But it's all just a game of advertising and algorithms that promote product placement, not necessarily the best solution for your child.

These types of treatment can't possibly consider the whole patient or get to the root cause of the symptoms.

Head and neck anatomy, nutrition, gut health, mental/emotional well-being, genetics, environment, generational trauma, body alignment, and more all play a big role in one's overall health. Plus, each patient reacts differently to all of those life variables. Like peeling back an onion, healthcare professionals must peel back the layers of contributing factors if we want to help patients.[4]

YOUR DOCTOR IS BIASED

According to an article by Stat News, forty percent of doctors report they're biased against certain groups of people when they come as patients. Weight, emotional problems, language disparities, and insurance coverage all play into triggering bias in physicians.[5]

Bias is defined as "a negative or positive idea a person has about someone or something. A person's bias can affect how they interact with people of certain groups."[6]

I'll be the first to admit that I have a bias regarding patients. My bias is a never-ending passion to educate.

Some patients don't like that. They don't want information; they want instructions. These families go elsewhere because I never tell someone what to do or force them.

So, what's a parent to do with all these twenty-first-century health problems? How can we make sure our children get the best health care? Now that we've uncovered some of the basics, let's dive deep and unearth the simple truth regarding our health.

PART TWO

PLAN

2

REJECT YOUR CURRENT REALITY

After my second heart surgery, I strove to be my healthiest, best version. I had become my own advocate and was well aware of my choices and their pros and cons. But let's fast forward.

Growing my dental practice and three young children only 15 months apart easily kept me busy. Still, I was eager for a fourth child. But I couldn't get pregnant. I suffered several miscarriages, including one late in my second trimester. Though uncommon, they left me heartbroken. While I tried to focus on my three healthy, beautiful children, I couldn't help feeling one person was missing.

Doctors encouraged me to take hormones, explore in vitro fertilization, and more, but I chose a more natural route. I began a holistic, life-changing, functional approach, and before we knew it, our sweet Eloise completed our family. My four kids are everything right with this world, and their existence motivates me to help improve and educate them to give them and their children a future full of potential.

Four healthy children, a strong marriage, and a thriving business—what more could I ask for? I felt on top of the world. Until my dermatologist presented me with a new diagnosis: cutaneous CD4-positive T-cell lymphoma—blood cancer.

My first reaction was, "You guys have to be kidding! I don't have time for this." I didn't have time for cancer. At the University of Texas Southwestern Medical Center, one of the top oncology hospitals in the country, they told me I would undergo surgery on New Year's Eve to remove the spot on my forehead that harbored these cells. They would try to be minimally invasive but start at my forehead and cut down the right side of my face to the bottom of my ear lobe. After the surgery, I'd have a facial scar and start chemo after the first of the year.

Somehow, though, the best thing for me seemed driven by my insurance benefits. During the discussions of both the date of the surgery and the timing of the chemo, insurance became the focus. How is that medically based? What if my medical insurance would not cover necessary procedures? Would the timelines or treatment plan change?

My oncologist oversimplified the explanation in the most empowering way to help me understand my choices. He explained that everybody has cancer cells circulating in their body. Cutaneous CD4 T-cell lymphoma happens when the body's environment becomes so toxic those cancer cells turn on.

I could have treated those toxic cancer cells with chemo and surgery, which many people must do. However, I was diagnosed so early that I had more options. First, I had to jump into the trenches and discover *why* my body had turned on these cancerous cells.

I examined every aspect of my life and found a list of felons.

High cortisol, or stress hormone, led the brigade, followed by tons of caffeine courtesy of my daily Italian expresso from our fancy machine. An internal critical commentary I wouldn't wish on anyone, coupled with toxic "mom friends" focused on gossip, contributed to the mess.

Sleep deprivation comes in a variety of forms. I burned the candle at both ends and traveled the world lecturing about this non-invasive treatment I offered in my office that I was so excited about that I wanted the entire world to know. One trip took me to Hong Kong to teach at the University. During my four-day stay, I slept a total of seven hours, then returned home to a full day seeing patients before my kids' soccer games. I loved it all, but my passion had turned manic, and my body was suffering. So little sunshine, always in a rush, ordering Uber Eats rather than cooking healthy meals—gee, I wonder where the toxicity came from?

Before Eloise arrived, we grew vegetables in a backyard garden; the kids picked tomatoes and lettuce when we wanted a salad. And our backyard chickens provided the eggs for breakfast. I needed to get back to that reality.

MOVE TO JOIN THE TRENCHES

In my practice; I focus on recognizing symptoms that stem from these altered realities we've become willing to live with. One area I concentrate on is sleep and breathing quality. This means airway maintenance for adults, but even more exciting is the more proactive, holistic approach for children. When we promote natural growth and development, kids don't turn into adults with breathing issues chasing symptoms that compromise their quality of life.

REJECT DIAGNOSES THAT DON'T MATCH YOUR LIFESTYLE

Not long ago; I had a four-year-old in my chair with a mouthful of cavities. His mother was in tears because her previous dentist criticized how he brushed his teeth and told her she fed him junk. But this kid ate an ideal gluten-free/sugar-free diet and had impeccable oral hygiene.

When this family joined our dental family, I affirmed their nutrition and oral hygiene habits and told them we needed to dig deeper to get more information. Mom was relieved and felt like she wasn't a failure.

We discovered the four-year-old's mouth breathing contributed to these cavities. This child was caught in a cortisol-induced oxygen desaturation event contributing to overall acidity. His saliva was so acidic that it was breaking down the enamel of his teeth, similar to the way a soda would. This mom carried shame and guilt for something she did not even understand. My heart broke for her and her child.

Between Instagram influencers, pediatricians, and your friends Google and Amazon, we have an overload of information and various alternate realities. Doctors need to sit down with patients, get back to the basics, and help patients create a healthy reality that works best for their particular family.

Make Sure Your Doctor is Biased Toward You

When looking for a provider that fits you and your family; it's important to find and match yourself with someone you trust who will give you all the information you need about your health. Anyone you work with should be open to all your questions. They should be supportive of the goals you have for your family.

If your goals are not to medicate long-term, the health provider you choose should have a plan for supplementation or a more natural route. Practitioners should spend time with you so you feel heard and addressed. They should have a like-minded team, so if they don't have the answer, they can refer you to someone who can help find the root cause of your issue.

Look for a humble, open person eager to learn about your situation. You want someone readily available. You should be able to call or reach out to them whenever you need help.

You and your provider need to be walking the same path and be committed to similar overall health goals. A doctor who smokes and then wants to talk about your heart may not be a good fit. A physician that fits your family will be working toward similar goals for his or her family and be open to speak to that as well. You'll find commonality and feel like they give you the best advice for your family.

3
REWIRE YOUR THINKING

IMMUNITY COMES FROM THE GUT

When we rewire our thinking, we must learn the difference between information and misinformation. The misinformation out there can be overwhelming, and many people need help knowing where to start. Often, we want an unrealistic quick fix.

Seventy percent of immunity is located in our guts.[14] If your gut isn't healthy and working the way it's supposed to, it will affect other areas in your body as well.

A great place to start rewiring your thinking and healing your gut with real credible information is on a website by Dr. Mark Hyman. He has many resources that will give you the tools you need to be successful, including a podcast, a newsletter, and more.

Dr. Weston Price, a Canadian dentist who lived in the early 1900s, offers these tips to begin gut healing:

- Exchange processed and ultra-processed foods for whole foods as much as possible.[15]

- Sleep.

- Use Castor oil packs and Epsom salt baths.

- Hydrate with proper minerals.

- Exercise regularly to increase the probiotic population and improve microbiome health.[15]

- Take a high-quality probiotic to rebalance your gut.[15]

Perhaps your family already does these things well. If so, it's time to dive even deeper. While gut health is essential, eliminating toxins becomes our number two strategy. Try some simple steps to help eliminate toxins daily:

- Skin: exfoliate, use non-toxic products, Epsom salt baths, and ionic foot baths.

- Gut: daily bowel movements, coffee enema, eating fiber-rich foods.

- Liver: eat cruciferous vegetables, castor oil packs.

- Lungs: exercise, deep diaphragmatic breathing, use a high-quality air filter.

- Lymphatics: rebounding, jump rope, massage, infrared sauna, dry brushing, vibration therapy, compression boots.

- Kidneys: hydrate, electrolytes, green juice.

- Mouth: oil pulling, tongue scraping, ozone oil.

- Mind: prayer, gratitude, meditation, positive attitude.

- Cellular: intermittent fasting, eliminate sugars and alcohol.

- Blood: exercise, infrared sauna, Nutritional IV therapy.

- Manage stress: getting outside, praying and meditating, deep breathing, contrast showers, and time with loved ones.

IS YOUR GUT TRUSTWORTHY?

In today's world, our attention is divided, making it difficult to complete our daily tasks. Social media, smartphones, multitasking, streaming videos, advertisements, and decision fatigue compete for our attention all day long. Did you know that, on average, people touch their phones 2,617 a day? [8] That's crazy! And while all these companies and devices fight for our attention, they also cause us to distrust ourselves. We need to get back to trusting our gut.

If you can't trust your gut, you have mixed emotions and feelings. Ninety percent of neurotransmitters come from the gut and are responsible for brain activity. That means ninety percent of the neurons that fire in your brain originate from your gut. It's like your second brain! That's where the phrase "trust your gut" comes from.

BACK TO BASICS: RESTORING HARMONY

It's ironic that when you're not feeling your best, you must be your strongest advocate. That's when you must push to find the answers.

So many of us are exhausted. There are so many decisions to make as parents—the right school, the right food, the right after-school activities. We eventually must find a point where we release the pressure and return to the basics: clean air, clean food, clean sleep, and clean thinking. All these things bring out the best version of us.

We obviously can't all move to a farm, have a cow, and raise chickens. Nor do we need personal trainers, private tutors, or many extra things.

Getting back to basics means we learn to align with our natural selves. Many people would be less overwhelmed if we got back to the basics.

I live in the city, drive a car, and wear clothes from the store. It would be cool if I could spin cotton, make my clothing, and avoid the toxins of fabrics, but I'm not doing that. However, we can take many little steps. Even drinking from a glass water bottle rather than plastic will improve your lifestyle.

Check out this list of things you can do right away with minimal effort:

Instead of this	Use this
Plastic water bottles	Glass water bottles
Aluminum antiperspirant deodorant	Nontoxic deodorant
Harsh chemical cleaners	Nontoxic cleaner- branch basics
Regular candles	Beeswax candles
Conventional meat	Pastured or grass-fed meat
Margarine and canola oil	Butter, Ghee, and Avocado Oil
Non-organic coffee	Organic coffee like Kion
Tide/conventional laundry products	Natural alternatives: Branch basics
Tap water	Filtered water
Nonstick cookware	Stainless steel or cast iron
Ibuprofen or Acetaminophen	Leefy Prana or Infammatone

INFORMATION VS. MISINFORMATION

It is important to understand the way the media controls us.

Instagram and Facebook algorithms watch our activity and send messages each time we log on. We need to differentiate between what the news and social media tell us is true and what is factual.

Where do you get your truth? Google, Amazon, and other sites use our searches and work with social media to feed us information based on that information. Backroom investors manipulate your thoughts and convince you to buy what they want to sell.

Do you need those pills? Or do you need some quiet time without social media? By choosing the latter, you are taking a step to rewire your thinking.

One of the most controversial topics I discuss with my patients revolves around non-healed root canals and their toxic effects on the rest of the body. By extracting the teeth from root canals that never healed and using ozone and platelet-rich fibrin (PRF), we have seen long-lasting symptoms like joint inflammation, sinus issues, and even breast cysts resolved. Unfortunately, these results get buried underneath studies that show how maintaining this dead tooth in your body is preferred despite an existing infection. It is a difficult conversation with a patient because it refutes what they have heard for so long.

WHERE ARE YOU GETTING YOUR TRUTH?

Rewiring your thinking about returning to basics and restoring your body doesn't have to be complicated.

I love the image of having a toxic bucket for your life. Whenever you do something toxic, you fill that bucket a little more. When someone drinks out of a water bottle, smokes cigarettes, stays up late with my friends gossiping, drinks a daily bottle of wine, or eats food full of GMOs, I picture the bucket filling. The bucket sounds like fun but not healthy. Still, to my astonishment, many people chose this lifestyle.

Eventually, one little thing will make the bucket overflow. You stay up too late on a Saturday, find yourself suddenly swollen with low energy, or discover a mass.

We need to create some non-negotiables as a counterbalance to keep our toxic bucket from overflowing. For example, for the next fourteen years, while my youngest is in school, I am going to live in a big city and drive an SUV so I can fit as many friends as we need in my car.

Maybe one day, I will live in Telluride, Colorado, where I can ride my bike or walk everywhere. Until then, I am a city girl who buys clothes off the rack. I will never make my own; that toxicity will always be in my bucket. To counter that bucket item, I'll only drink from glass containers and spend the extra money to get grass-fed meat and non-toxic skin products. Unless we're extremely disciplined, we'll never empty the bucket entirely, but we can create some healthy practices that open the space to keep the toxicity from overflowing. When I sleep well, eat, drink, and think clean, I ensure the bucket stays balanced.

I was born competitive, so it's difficult for me to have clean, supportive thoughts about myself all of the time. High achievers relentlessly push themselves, and I have to be my biggest fan, right? That's who I am, and I'm never going to change. But I must balance that by surrounding myself with friends who offset my own negative commentary.

I married the perfect man for me. He is relaxed, supportive, and makes me laugh daily. His dedication to our family is unwavering, and he is a consistent example of what is truly important. When I suggested we eat healthier and hired a raw food chef to live in her camper in our driveway, he was completely on board. And on those days I vent to him about business issues or distracting gossip, he always answers with the ideal "forget 'em."

I rewired my thinking as I became my advocate, and it's a joy to watch my patients change their perspective and take hold of their health future.

4

REWRITE YOUR STORY

When I met Nick, he was a fifty-year-old "loser" deadbeat who had lost custody of his children, and his wife divorced him because of his addictions.

I couldn't condone or excuse his poor behavior. But his past didn't mean he could never change his story to something more positive. Over time, he had lost the idea of what success meant, which for him, was providing for his family.

He knew they were bad choices. This divorced father of two used cocaine every morning and drank a handle of vodka every night. As an entrepreneur in the carpet business, his income directly relied on his daytime productivity. He needed the uppers to get him out of bed and the downers to knock him out so he could function the next day. It was the only way he could sleep at night.

Nick was not a wild and crazy party person; he was simply doing anything he could to function. But his undiagnosed breathing problems caused him to lose his wife, children, and business before a toothache brought him into my office.

We made simple changes to Nick's upper and lower jaws with the wear of an oral appliance so he could breathe without interruption through the night.

After Nick began rewriting his story, he realized he needed to figure out a way to get his family back. He wanted to make decisions his family would be proud of. So, Nick checked into a thirty-day rehab facility to focus on his sleep and beat his addictions. Nick just celebrated eighteen months sober and has joint custody of his two beautiful children. Now he is working to rebuild his business with focus and intention.

He still has some work to do with the children, for sure. But suppose he continues to rewrite his story and believes that he's not a deadbeat loser but a loving caretaker who made bad decisions to compensate and survive; his family will find hope and empowerment.

AS A MOM, YOU CAN REWRITE YOUR FAMILY'S STORY

Many moms share a similar reality. Hubby works and travels a lot. She stays home tending children, the house, and maybe even a job outside the home too. So Mom is exhausted from her very busy and full life.

I have four kids, own a business, and wake up clear-headed every morning, ready to attack the day. Does that surprise you? Most people think it's impossible to raise children, take care of patients, and also feel good and feel happy. I reached this point only by rewriting my own story.

I had three kids in three years. (Not intentionally—we wanted children, but not necessarily that close together.) In the six years before I got pregnant with the fourth, I had three miscarriages, including the second-trimester miscarriage I mentioned earlier.

The traditional advice was to let your body heal and try again. But my gut instinct told me something else needed adjusting. I was thirty-five, too young to be considered late-stage or advanced maternal age, yet, I knew I needed to find out more.

I examined my life and realized I woke up each day acting like an anorexic Cookie Monster. Each morning, I started with coffee, then worked all day without lunch. At the end of the work day, I arrived home carrying the emotional baggage of my patients. After serving my three children a healthy dinner of salmon and quinoa, we'd have a blissful time of reading stories, and I'd tuck them in. By that time, I'd be so tired I would have a cookie from the pantry before I crashed into bed, where I would work for three or four more hours before I fell asleep. I can't tell you the number of times I fell asleep holding my phone or my laptop.

I was exhausted, emotionally drained, and sustaining myself with easy-to-grab processed food and cookies.

Looking back, I can't help but wonder why I didn't sit and eat dinner with my family. My children would have loved for me to sit down and eat with them. They didn't mind dirty dishes in the sink. They wanted me to set an extra plate. Today, it seems insane that I didn't.

I think it was an issue of low self-worth. Like so many moms, I sacrificed myself to live out my ideal narrative: I make wonderful healthy meals and provide a clean home for my family. At the same time, I completely disregarded my own needs. The beautiful facade allowed me to wear *busy* as a badge of honor. It sounds bizarre, but I think it's common.

I was caught up in this toxic identity of the perfect mom. Without proper sleep or eating habits, I may as well have been the carpet salesman addicted to drugs. Espresso every morning and wine every night—of course, my body wasn't ready to sustain a new life.

Once I decided to rewrite my story, I started an elimination diet to decrease inflammation and add mineral water to my daily routine. Tony Robbins' passionate talks replaced the news or audio parenting books on the drive home. And on other days, I jammed to Justin Bieber full blast. It seemed silly, but it wasn't.

Not long after I rewrote my story with healthy thoughts, food, drinks, and sleep, I became pregnant with our fourth child. I felt so grateful. However, sixty days into the pregnancy, the danger zone for a miscarriage passed, and I started slacking.

As I began to plan my maternity leave, I found ways to overschedule myself so I could see all my patients before I had my baby. Plus, I wanted to spend quality time with all my kids, so I planned special one-on-one trips with them before this new baby arrived.

After sweet Eloise's birthday, I got the call about my cord blood that I attempted to bank for future medical issues if they were to arise. Pregnancy assaulted my immune system in a big way. It caused inflammation and turned on those cells. The second cord blood test came back positive for toxic cells again. I felt as if I had destroyed my unborn child's future.

I felt like a hypocrite. I had been treating my patients and advising them on how to live well while burning the candle at both ends and living another.

Ozone treatments to sterilize my blood and kill unhealthy cells again became part of my life. Rewriting my story again included red light therapy, saunas, exercise, and increasing my water intake with proper minerals to support my detox reactions. My children attended many of these activities with me, so we had quality time while doing something healthy. Fortunately, the body is miraculous. Despite the abuse we put through, the body can always heal.

KEEP REWRITING—OVER AND OVER

I had to rewrite my story again after my lymphoma diagnosis. So many questions and assumptions began to fill the pages. What would happen if I had a scar on my face? What about my lymphatic system? I already struggled with my vision. What if the surgery caused headaches that affected my hearing? What would chemo do to my hormones? Would this affect menopause? What would my health look like five, ten, or twenty years from now?

I want to make decisions today that I still feel confident about in twenty or thirty years. I was done making compensations for my health. It was time to fill the pages of my story with my choice of words.

I didn't want chemo, and I didn't want surgery. I decided to return to being the healthiest and best version of myself and advocate for myself again. I wanted to jump into a functional space and treat my blood cancer with alternative therapies.

I'm happy to say I'm almost five and a half years in remission. Western doctors said, "This is a miracle; you're so lucky." And maybe that's true—it is a miracle, and I am lucky. But I also intervened to help heal myself. Part of that included a clean life—no inflammatory gluten, dairy, or sugar. Plus, I gave proper oxygenation to all the vital processes of my body so I could achieve healing and detox during my sleep.

I needed clean thoughts. What did I do to ensure I had them? I created new boundaries in every relationship of my life. I focused on what I wanted to do rather than what I thought I should do. People were not always comfortable with my new boundaries, but I stuck with them. I downloaded the Headspace app and listened for five minutes in the morning. I read books that positively influenced my internal dialogue and only watched shows that made me laugh. (Thank you, Bravo!).

I eliminated toxic relationships.

Long-time friendships don't always mean healthy relationships. I created a much healthier environment by eliminating or limiting my exposure to those individuals. I found little tricks, and I returned to the basics. Whenever I waivered, I called my best friend Niki, who lives an honest and transparent life I try to emulate.

After having a bone marrow biopsy, we discovered the cancer was isolated to my blood, which was great news. I felt optimistic about changing my lifestyle so I did not have to continue to compensate. I began ozone IV therapy to make sure my cells were getting the proper oxygen. This process required that I be hooked up to a high-dose ozone machine that would draw my blood and pump it full of supercharged oxygen. The machine would kill the virus and bacteria in the blood and then return it to my body. Ozone therapy kills unhealthy cells and pumps up healthy cells, so it's a win-win. I worked with a doctor who used a holistic approach to help me navigate alternative treatment options, including hyperbaric oxygen chambers, ionic foot baths, red light therapy, and saunas.

Does that mean everyone with cancer can undergo ozone therapy and avoid surgery? Absolutely not. But everyone should be able to feel empowered with options and alternative routes to support their health. Many people have the same blood cancer I had. They have surgery, go through chemo, live, thrive, and are happy. I'm happy for those people, but that was not the right decision for me. Neither way is wrong, but we are entitled to understand the pros and cons of both sides.

Because the cells in our body turnover every thirty days, I retested my blood after the first month. Guess what? Those cancerous cells were gone. This motivated me to live a healthier life. Living a healthy lifestyle is a delicate balance we're trying to achieve. Rather than focusing on the negative, I prefer to look at everything in moderation.

EVERYTHING IN MODERATION–MOVED

Rewriting your story doesn't mean your story is written in stone. It may need to be revised again when another big life event comes your way. For instance, I've written my story that I usually eat, drink, think, and sleep healthy. Then other times, I know I'll be traveling for a weekend and eating out a lot, and my schedule will be off. No worries, I'll drink a lot of water, get a Vitamin C IV, and eat healthy leading up to my trip to balance out the toxic behavior I can't avoid over the weekend. Everything is in moderation, including moderation. If we strive to make eighty percent of our lifestyle healthy, we will notice the difference in how we feel. That is the view that serves us best. Be your own advocate. Rewrite your story and allow it to have enough flexibility so you can live your life.

5

REKINDLE YOUR FIGHT

Have you seen *The Lion King*? This story offers so many tremendous lessons. Spoiler alert: Mufasa dies, and Simba runs away from his kingdom because he's been convinced he caused his father's death. Negativity controls Simba's thoughts.

Rafiki eventually found the prince and reminded him that he was the child of the King, his dad's spirit lived on in him, and he needed to return home to take his rightful place. Rafiki finally persuaded Simba to fight back by reinforcing his identity as the future king.

Most people hate coming to the dentist for fillings and other dental work. Plus, they think it's too expensive. I've found that patients' perspectives improve if I change the narrative to, "Hey, this should be pain-free." And "We should never have to do this again because we're treating the root causes."

OVERWHELMED PATIENTS NEED AN ADVOCATE

Seven-year-old Liam came into our office with Attention Deficit Hyperactivity Disorder (ADHD). During his first visit, he ran in and punched a hole in my waiting room wall. He shocked the entire staff.

My discussion with his mother turned to the reason Liam had cavities. Yes, every kid can brush and floss better, but Liam's problems stemmed from something more. His cavities were located between the teeth near where the salivary ducts deposit spit. I suspected he had increased acidity in his saliva. Teeth bathed in that saliva day and night, combined with the oral hygiene of a seven-year-old, created a mouth-perfect storm of cavities.

Liam needed someone to help him rewrite his story, change his identity, and ultimately rekindle his fight for health. I started by telling him he was amazing, brave, and strong. Four months of wearing new night mouth appliances, making dietary changes, and doing yoga to improve his headspace, a child with a totally different demeanor came to his next appointment. His body no longer needed to compensate as the series of appliances that we introduced resolved the poor oral habits he was using to compensate in an effort to promote the natural growth and development of this child so that he could breathe and sleep efficiently. Every child in our dental family is evaluated for this approach as we know these appliances can resolve the issue rather than just putting a bandaid on the symptom.

Today's world prefers quick fixes for symptoms. I could have just filled Liam's cavities. But that wouldn't have fixed the root of the problem. Liam needed someone to advocate for him, to tell him brushing and flossing wouldn't be enough, and help him see that even his ADHD symptoms could be controlled better.

Advocacy rekindles the fight. Whether you act as your own or your child's advocate, when you have the knowledge to make better decisions, you will feel empowered to battle and control your own health.

Advocates Fight for Their Children

What if we investigated the root cause of mouth breathing instead of rushing into surgery? What if we could teach them to use their nose to breathe and eliminate the symptoms?

I know a very sweet boy named Luke. At four, he began punching other children at school. At the parent-teacher conference, the teacher didn't want to discuss his obvious anger problems but instead told Luke's mom she believed he had a speech issue. His mom understood every word, and Luke was a smart kid, but when he talked about dinosaurs and ninjas. Frustrated, he punched them. It wasn't an anger issue; it was a speech issue. Luke was upset that the other kids didn't understand his warnings about dinosaurs and ninjas coming to take over the world! (Luke definitely didn't lack imagination).

If your tongue can't go into the correct position, or you're fighting to breathe appropriately, you will compensate with your speech. Even with good medical insurance, families spend thousands of dollars on speech therapy and still don't always get the clarity they're looking for.

When a space exists between the two front teeth, orthodontists and parents are eager to close it. But we need to ask why that space, or diastema, exists in the first place. Metal braces have been used for decades to close that space, but adding the braces can put the tongue in jail. They push the tongue back into the airway. I can't tell you how many thirty and forty-somethings have beautiful smiles created with metal braces that come with a compromised airway blocked by the tongue. Metal retainers glued to the back of their front teeth keep them in place. This sets them up for a lifetime of compensations, like grinding teeth, popping and clicking in their joints, and muscular issues, such as weak lip muscles, potentially leading to Botox and fillers.

Research links metal retainer bar and cement to disturbed thyroid function and hormonal levels. But without that piece of metal, their tongue thrust would open that space again. Oh, but they have beautiful smiles! And their bodies have to compensate to maintain it.

Doctors treat all the complications, but if the tongue could function the way it is supposed to, they would be able to breathe and not have these complications. I prefer a more proactive approach by resolving improper tongue function before aligning teeth when children are younger.

Proper tongue posture and proper breathing in children help promote the growth of the upper and lower jaw through the use of removable oral appliances. This allows us to avoid being reactive using extra forces like metal braces or expanders. When the jaw grows naturally, the tongue falls forward and out of the airway, and we change the patient's future. At my office, we call it the Super Health program!!

CHANGE TODAY FOR A NEW TOMORROW

Rekindling your fight for health means that your present circumstances won't have to define you.

You're capable of seizing your destiny and fighting for a better tomorrow.

A twelve-year-old who sucked his thumb visited my office. *I can't help but suck my thumb. I need to stop. Eww, the germs!* He thought this every time he sucked his thumb.

I switched his narrative by telling him, "Hey, you're a genius. I'm so impressed that you figured out how to suck your thumb like that. Most people aren't as smart as you. You are amazing. Let's stop for a second and celebrate how amazingly intelligent you are. I cannot wait to see what you decide to do when you grow up." The demeanor of this child changed completely as the shame he felt seemed to melt away.

But why did I praise his thumb-sucking? His thumb in his mouth advanced his mandible, which trained his jaw to move forward and allowed him to breathe better by bringing his tongue out of his airway. It's the same reason Michael Jordan has his tongue out while flying through the air during one of his famous slam dunks on my husband's garage poster. When you breathe better, you perform better because you have more oxygen.

This boy didn't suck his thumb because he was insecure. He had inadvertently figured out that bringing his jaw forward allowed his tongue to get out of the way, and he could breathe better.

As I said earlier, your nose is supposed to filter, purify, and humidify the air before it sends it throughout the body. But air quality is just as important as well as quantity. If either is compromised, the body will have to compensate; This is so critical to overall health that I discuss it with every patient.

The instinct to breathe is stronger than any other. This boy feels ashamed, gets made fun of, and refuses to have sleepovers. His social life suffers because he is smart enough to figure out how to breathe.

Despite his superior intelligence, we needed to find something else to help him stay oxygenated. I wanted it to be something people wouldn't misunderstand or cause him to feel more shame.

We discovered he had an anterior tongue thrust. Every time he swallowed, his tongue came forward instead of to the roof of his mouth. Normally, the tongue goes to the palate about 3000 times a day, putting pressure on the upper jaw to help expand it. However, if you've been bringing your tongue forward since infancy to bring your tongue out of your airway, you never put pressure on that bone. As a result, that upper jaw stays small and doesn't grow right. Eventually, the upper jaw will have a vaulted arch, the tongue will end up in the wrong position, and breathing will be hampered.

We gave this young man an oral appliance to bring his lower jaw forward while he slept. Through orthopedic myofunctional therapy (a program that corrects improper use of the tongue and facial muscles)[13], we brought that lower jaw forward. We retrained his tongue so he could breathe better. Not only did he change the poor oral habit that contributed to the problem, but he was also able to catch up so he could continue to develop appropriately.

Other professionals had recommended cutting off part of the back of his tongue. This would have opened his airway. But the root cause was not too big a tongue; it was too small a jaw.

He had the hardest time putting on the corrective device the first time. He gagged on it. I told him, "Just try wearing this for a bit while I talk with your mom."

I began speaking with his mom, but I knew he was listening. I told his mom I could tell he was extremely smart and strong. "He's been able to compensate and keeps himself healthy." As I spoke, I watched him focus more on what I was saying. I knew he just needed his thinking rewired. I wanted him to hear how capable he was of wearing the appliance. No one feels motivated to change when they feel weak.

Within five minutes, he had the device in his mouth and started breathing easily through his nose. He wholeheartedly agreed to take it home and try it. It was a nighttime appliance, but I knew he needed a little extra practice before he tried to sleep with it. So I suggested he try wearing it while he played an hour of video games daily. He thought I was awesome, as his mom restricts screen time to 1 hour on weekends only! We broke his thumb habit within six days because he retold his story in his brain. He wasn't weak. He could conquer anything.

I talked to the boy's mother a few years after his treatment was complete. A friend had been made fun of for sucking her thumb during math class in high school. He stood up for her by telling his classmates that she was probably smarter than all of them because she had figured out how to breathe and think better. He proved his theory by showing everyone the A she had earned on her calculus test while everyone else relied on the curve.

Empowering a young boy to defend a classmate for something she couldn't help—I call leaving the world a better place than I found it.

We broke his thumb habit, and he has had dry beds ever since. He has a social life and sleepovers. He retold the positive identity story in his brain that rekindled his fight and changed his tomorrow. He also changed the tomorrow for the girl in his math class and gave her the confidence to fight for herself. I can only hope she changes the tomorrow for someone else. And that is ultimately how we make this big world a better place—changing each other's tomorrows for the better.

These stories motivate me to continue on this educational journey with my patients. The boy's math genius friend showed up in my office a few weeks later, and we helped her. She is now an engineering major at MIT and tutors low-income students in math. Take that thumb sucker, shamers!

FOCUS GOES—ENERGY FLOWS

Tony Robbins says, "Where focus goes, energy flows. And where energy flows, whatever you're focusing on grows."[16]

We structure our lives according to what we center our focus on.

Sometimes, my patients or their parents are caught in a rut. They tell themselves they (or their children) are sick or weak. And because they continue to focus their energy there, it quickly becomes their identity.

By altering our focus, we can change our identities into something positive and rekindle the fight we have within ourselves to fight for our own and our children's health.

6

RESEARCH YOUR OPTIONS

Sadly, children of the twenty-first century commonly experience ADHD, bedwetting, irritability, allergies, anxiety, headaches, and inflammation. And despite all the advancements in medicine in the last hundred years, the current treatments simply put a bandage on the problem. A diagnosis of ADHD, anxiety, or headaches immediately calls for medication. Tonsil inflammation requires surgery. As Taylor Swift says in one of my favorite songs, "bandaids don't fix bullet holes."

It's time to begin asking *why* these kids have ADHD. *Why* are they anxious? *Why* are their tonsils inflamed? By looking at the whole patient, we can find the root cause; otherwise, they will need to compensate for the rest of their lives. When your child shows symptoms, it's important to advocate for them and research all options for treatment. One size doesn't fit all in medical treatments.

Many times, lifestyle and home routine changes make for a great beginning. For instance, sometimes children's poor behavior, including irritability and ADHD symptoms, is simply a reaction to allergies. When your child has trouble breathing due to a dust allergy, they lose sleep at night and experience overall discomfort during the day. Even adults don't behave well when they feel tired or uncomfortable.

Dr. Benjamin Feingold, a pediatric allergist, theorized diet had a connection to child behavior. In the 1970s, he used restricted diets to treat allergies and noted a significant improvement in the child's behavior. Dr. Feingold's theory pioneered behavioral studies linking allergy and diet. [9]

Allergy-related behavioral issues easily get misdiagnosed as attention deficit disorder (ADD) or attention deficit hyperactivity disorder (ADHD) with an accompanying medication prescription. Unfortunately, that means the food allergy continues, perhaps doing more damage than simply causing bad behavior.

Simple changes at home can help you get back to the basics:

- Install an air filter or negative ionizer for your home.

- Get a water filtration device (even refrigerator-filtered water is better than public water supply).

- Leave your cell phone in another room at night.

- Turn the TV off before you go to bed.

- Utilize the Headspace app to clear your mind.

- Work out earlier in the day instead of late at night.

- Eliminate high-inflammatory foods like gluten, sugar, and dairy from your diet.

- Supplement your diet with a multivitamin or glutathione (it's hard to get the minerals and nutrients you need from our current foods).

- Taking a melatonin supplement before bedtime to help regulate your sleep. (Our brain is confused by all the time we spend on screens. Are we supposed to be awake, or are we supposed to be asleep? With supplementations, you can help your body get back to working the way it's supposed to).

- Go outside during the middle of the day to get some sun and natural Vitamin D.

- Use a nasal lavage like a Neti Pot or Nasal Pure. (Mouth breathing causes tonsils and adenoids to filter air triggering an inflammatory response in your lungs. Nasal lavages neutralize the acidic inflammation with salt).

- Oral appliance therapy for kids (like our Super Health program!) helps promote the natural growth and development of their upper and lower jaw by letting the tongue work the way it's supposed so they can learn to breathe through their nose.

- Utilize infrared light to decrease inflammation.

- Ionic footbaths are salt water with an electrical current that pulls toxins out of your body.

Many patients complete our thirty-day reset program and feel remarkably better and tremendously grateful. Regret and anger often follow as they realize they have been living a compromised life because no one told them the simplicity of natural healing.

The body is perfect. It's miraculous and can heal if we know how to help it. A bit of research and education will allow us to restore our bodies to their factory settings.

Asking the Right Questions Makes All the Difference

I wish you could meet my teenage patient, Laura. She earns straight A's, has many friends, and loves athletics. Laura rescues dogs, writes poetry, has loving parents, and enjoys a beautiful life. Despite all these positives, Laura has never truly felt good. She always felt exhausted, and I suspected she never got restorative sleep. With her teenage hormones already out of control, Laura also suffered emotional dysregulation—the inability to control or regulate emotional responses—because of sleep-disordered breathing. As a result, she often felt the highest of highs and lowest of lows.

When she came to me three years ago, I noticed the cut marks on her arms. These conversations are never comfortable, but we have to broach the subject. If I don't say anything, the child may think it's unimportant to me, and if everybody is uncomfortable, no one will have the conversation. That child may never get the help they need.

I wanted Laura to know my office was a safe place. I gave her my cell phone number and promised to keep it confidential. Five minutes after she left, I got a text asking if we could talk.

She returned and said, "Listen, I know I should be happy," which resonated with me. She continued, "I'm miserable. I don't sleep. I'm nervous all the time. I have so much anxiety."

We learned more when she did a home sleep test. Our research showed that Laura breathes beautifully while sitting up; however, her nighttime oxygen desaturation sent her into a cortisol-induced sympathetic state.

A child needs restful, uninterrupted sleep for their growing body to rest, repair, and detox before the next day. If that doesn't happen consistently, it can contribute to these anxious feelings that Laura was negatively expressing when she cut herself.

I told her, "Laura, I understand why you feel so low. I am grateful that you trust me, and I am eager to help you find a way to feel better."

Because Laura was self-harming, I told her I had to inform her parents. She was relieved and upset at the same time. She confessed that her parents knew but didn't know how to make her feel better either. I related to that feeling of helplessness from Laura and her parents much more than I liked.

I told Laura and her parents about Nick. They didn't immediately understand the connection. I explained how his story demonstrated the importance of restful sleep and consistent breathing.

Laura and her parents stared at me wide-eyed after listening to Nick's story. Her dad had tears in his eyes as he realized Laura's problems went beyond her mental well-being. I told Laura she was God's child and perfect the way she was, but we had to get to the root cause to make her feel better. I assured her she hadn't done anything to cause the problem. Simply telling somebody, "Hey, it's not your fault; we can make it better," makes a huge difference in how they approach their healing.

Three years later, Laura is functioning beautifully. Her mom tells every patient in the office I saved her daughter's life. They usually roll their eyes and ask, "How does a dentist save your life?"

Laura's healing had nothing to do with her teeth and everything to do with her breathing and sleeping. I just asked the right questions and researched to present her with the right tools. The result was a young girl empowered to live the best version of herself.

Most kids are eager to please; they want to feel better. I tear up every time I see the beautiful Laura enter a room, knowing her future, much like mine, could have been so different if we hadn't addressed the root cause.

7

RENEW YOUR HOPE

I've already shared some stories that should give you hope for your future. What has happened to these patients can become your reality, too. You and your family no longer need to live without hope. It might take asking a lot of questions and researching practitioners until you find the one that fits your story the best, but as you take control of your health, you should begin to feel renewed hope.

CREATING HEALTHY HABITS RENEWS HOPE

Creating health in our lives takes a lifetime of cultivating good habits. When we get off track, we need a healthy habit to get us back on track and pay off some of that unhealthy habit debt. We pay back the debt with good sleep and hygiene habits. We can put our phones away at night, turn off the TV, set the thermostat to a cooler temperature, invest in bamboo sheets, wash with a chemical-free detergent, and wear comfortable pajamas. All these things are important.

I call this bad habit debt oxygen debt. Every new patient completes a screening evaluating their overnight oxygen saturation and breathing ability in my practice. With this screening, we can determine if we can help them or if they need a referral to a like-minded provider.

A nap once or twice a week can help pay back that debt. But you need to ensure you and your bed partner don't disturb each other. Schedule naps as seriously as you schedule meetings at work or sports practices. Adjusting to your new healthy lifestyle may make you feel a bit worse before turning the corner.

TAKING CONTROL OF YOUR HEALTH RENEWS HEALTH

One of my patients worked with a fertility clinic after having trouble getting pregnant naturally. She had followed every recommendation except navigating the sleep portion of her health. Plagued with unexplained adrenal fatigue and Hashimoto's disease, she discovered interrupted sleep caused her oxygen levels to drop, triggering a cortisol reaction.

Four months after she corrected her sleep by stabilizing her oxygen, she naturally became pregnant. It's incredible what the body can do.

A private school in Dallas caters to children who have severe ADHD. They're incredibly smart, but they have diagnosed learning differences. With parental consent, I offered a complimentary screening with first graders to check for signs of sleep-disordered breathing. Thirty-seven out of fifty-two had a sleep issue. We presented potential treatment options from those consultations, including oral appliance therapy in my office or other services with trusted, like-minded providers.

At least twenty of these children matriculated back into conventional classrooms without being disruptive. These children no longer needed the private school's special accommodations to be successful. The children's hope was restored.

We all need hope to unlock our full potential and become the best version of ourselves.

Nick rewired his thinking and rewrote his story. Then with renewed hope, he fought to get his family back. Laura went from self-mutilation to self-confidence; a boy who sucked his thumb much longer than he would have liked moved from insecurity to joy. Liam changed his story and renewed his hope. His reality of ADHD and disruptive behavior is behind him. He's now in school, has friends, and played the role of Prince Charming in his class musical.

When I woke up from my first surgery, the doctor told me that shortness of breath, an enlarged liver, and a swollen face and legs were my new normal. He told me to deal with it, and I felt weak. But like the others, I rejected that reality rewired my thinking, rewrote my story, rekindled my fight, and renewed my hope.

8

REIMAGINE YOUR OTHER SIDE

I never want someone to feel the depth of sadness, hopelessness, or helplessness I felt that day waiting in Dr. Fraser's office. That experience taught me to continue searching for answers and reimagine the other side of any situation.

The other side of my mishandled heart surgery spurs my hope. I run a business I love and have patients who trust and value me. My team of employees brings me joy as I watch them eager to be the best versions of themselves and provide for our patients. I adore my tremendous family—my husband, who is my life partner and loves me in a way I always dreamed, and four beautiful, imperfect children who motivate me to understand our world better. I have the privilege of traveling the world with these people I love and experiencing adventures bigger than I could envision. That's my other side.

I'm happy—truly happy—on the inside. My other side won't look like yours, but that's the beauty of reimagining.

BRINGING OUT YOUR BEST SELF ON THE OTHER SIDE

When I started lecturing and teaching dentists how to use the appliances I work with, someone asked me why I do what I do. I answered, "If we can help kids be the best versions of themselves, maybe they will help us later and make a difference in this world."

At my weakest, I wasn't my true self, and now I'm beyond grateful to get back to the real me. I want to help kids and their families get there, to educate them and help them understand they can have better if they want it. You can wake up with a clear head tomorrow and suddenly be energetic. How could that change life?

At a party last Christmas, I overserved myself champagne and danced the night away. The next day, I felt the effects. I parented from bed, we skipped church, and my kids watched TV all day. The entire day was exhausting. My thoughts returned to the Sunday before when my family and I ate breakfast together, went hiking, and enjoyed a beautiful day together.

I realized that some of the parents in my practice are parenting in a hungover state every day. They walk around exhausted, chronically sick, and so unhappy that they use alcohol to feel better. Then the next day, they feel worse. If they could just learn to reject their current reality and begin the steps toward empowerment, they, too, could reimagine the other side.

Every parent has the opportunity to save their children from a future they need not experience. When we make proactive, holistic, and non-invasive decisions while they're growing and developing, we save them from a future that leaves them either exhausted and chronically sick or full of disease. My goal is to give them hope to reimagine their other side.

PART THREE

PLEDGE

9

JOIN THE MOVEMENT IN THE TRENCHES

In my early twenties, I thought I was at the pinnacle of life. That all came to a screeching stop with my botched heart surgery. I trusted medical providers to make decisions for me that, looking back, weren't things I would have chosen if I had been given the appropriate information. That experience created a passion within me to make sure everyone knows their options when it comes to their health. I want to teach people how to advocate not only for themselves but also for their children.

The majority of mothers long to do the absolute best for their kids. However, with all the information and misinformation, trying to navigate how to make the best decisions for our children for their health can be overwhelming.

Getting back to the basics of breathing, swallowing, and sleeping correctly will amazingly make many of these outward symptoms disappear. Today children compensate with seemingly "normal" things like mouth breathing, teeth grinding, thumb sucking, or bedwetting. There's a whole host of compensations healthy kids live with in order to survive. But we want more for our children. With the proper information and rewired thinking, we can rewrite their stories and help their little bodies work how they should. They would no longer have to compensate.

IN THE TRENCHES, WE WRITE NEW REALITIES

In the mom groups I join, we talk a lot about what our kids are going through. We share stories and support one another. Many stories remind me just because it's common doesn't mean it's normal. Just because more than one mother shares the same concerns or symptoms doesn't mean we need to accept that as the reality for our kids.

Realizing your children deserve better than what's being accepted as normal can be empowering. Our kids deserve to function and be the best version of themselves, but we must sift through the common tales we tell each other. When we get into the trenches as moms, we can figure out a way forward.

WHAT WE'RE CURRENTLY DOING IN THE TRENCHES

I am so proud of the culture we have built at Central Dentist. We strive to empower patients to take control of their health by addressing root causes rather than treating symptoms. These empowered patients refer their friends and family. Surrounding myself with people like this all day is a dream. The old saying, "If you love what you do, then you never work a day in your life," rings true as I continue to build a practice full of motivated, like-minded people who teach me as much as I share with them.

YOU DESERVE THE BEST

We founded my office's Super Health program on the same philosophy as functional medicine. We offer holistic myofunctional and dental therapy to guide patients along a path to sustainable oral health and wellness.

The program offers the culmination of the most advanced, evidence-based therapies to provide our patients with the care they need to heal, optimize their oral and dental health, and educate them on how to maintain optimal wellness for a lifetime.[7]

However, I've recognized over the years that while this philosophy and practice makes perfect sense to me and has been proven effective over and over again, one of our biggest challenges in providing this care is providing this paradigm shift for patients who are unaware of the importance of whole body health. They don't understand that "common" does not necessarily mean healthy.

I identify these kinds of patients when they say things like, "This approach worked for me, so it'll work for my kids," or "This is what everyone else is doing, so I'm sure it's right." I try to empathize and start where that parent is at the moment—mentally, emotionally, and physically—and speak to that. Other times I can't stand by and watch. I end up saying something like: "Just because the majority of the adult US population is obese, does that mean it's healthy?" Or in moments when I'm feeling extra feisty, "Remember for so many decades when everyone thought it was 'normal' to smoke cigarettes, including pregnant women? Just because it was so commonplace did not inherently make it healthy." [4]

You may have excuses for neglecting your health. Perhaps you're a working mom with four kids. But you deserve the best too. You wouldn't allow your child to get away with that. Taking care of health is not exclusive to children. Let's stop using what everyone considers normal as an excuse and change the narrative surrounding our health.

I urge you to join the movement once you put down this book. It's time to reject your reality, rewire your intuition, rekindle your fight, rewrite your story, research your options, renew your hope, and reimagine your other side. Join those of us who are aiming to change too.

If you're struggling with where to start, I encourage you to take the Happy Mom Pledge at *Mother.ly/life/the-happy-mom-pledge* where you will promise always to give yourself grace when you stumble.

It's time to take back your health and your life. I know you're already doing awesome things as a mom;

otherwise, you'd never have picked up a book that might help you be better. Motherhood puts us in the trenches whether we want to be there or not. I just don't want you to be there alone.

ACKNOWLEDGMENTS

Along this journey, I learned that if I blame someone for all of the bad, I must also thank them for all of the good that came from this negative event. So my sincerest thank you to the doctors who gave me the wrong diagnosis and then told me I would never physically be able to have children, the friends who ditched me, the other moms who think I am too crunchy for happy hour, and the brainwashed egomaniacs who think their way is the only way. Your negativity and presumed limitations have lit a fire within me that continues to burn brighter every day.

To Mom and Dad- I lack the words to truly describe my gratitude for both of you, from my lovely childhood to being active grandparents to my four kids. Thank you for supporting me exactly as I am and finding my voice and the message I wanted to share. I can't imagine it has always been easy to be my parents, but you did everything right, and I am forever grateful to both of you.

To Will and Beth- Thank you for your support during all my recoveries. I don't remember how many family holidays or events I ruined being sick or recovering but thank you for always being patient and present.

To my very bestest friend in the whole wide world- Niki- I am so grateful for your friendship. Most of my favorite and most hilarious stories of my life involve you. Thank you for being the most amazingly loyal and understanding friend a girl could ever ask for.

To the twinkles in my eye- Franny, Vinny, Gino, and Eloise- I am so proud of all 4 of you. I love you more than anything. You are my reason for being in the trenches and figuring out how to help you become the very best version of yourself. If you read this book, I hope you understand me better and why my "work" is also very important to me. Balancing being a mom and dentist is not easy, and I hope this gives you insight into why both are so very important to me. I love you the most and forever.

To Jimbo- In sickness and in health. You showed me the meaning of those vows before we even got married. You have always been the most careful with my heart, and I do not know what I did to deserve you, but I will love you forever. Thank you for always being there and loving me no matter how I showed up.

ABOUT THE AUTHOR

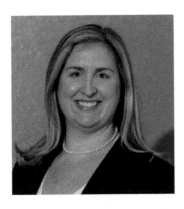

Dr. Jill Ombrello and her team at Central Dentist offer diverse services, including early intervention orthodontics, periodontal therapies, airway evaluation, ceramic biocompatible implants, ozone treatments, TMD therapy, and cosmetic smile makeovers. She founded Onsite Dentists of Texas, PLLC, which accommodates patients incapable of traveling to a traditional facility by bringing comprehensive care to them. As a passionate advocate for improving the lives of children, Dr. Ombrello specializes in sleep-disordered breathing and habit correction for children aged two to twelve. Learn more at CentralDentist.com.

NOTES

1. "New research finds 'Dr. Google' is almost always wrong." Neuroscience News. May 17, 2020. https://neurosciencenews.com/dr-google-wrong-16408/#:~:text=Summary%3A%20Turning%20to%20Google%20for,one%2Dthird%20of%20the%20time.&text=Many%20people%20turn%20to%20%27Dr

2. Spry, Terry, et al. "VERIFY: How accurate are WebMD results?" WKYC Studios. September 13, 2019. https://www.wkyc.com/article/news/verify/verify-how-accurate-are-webmd-results/507-d455712d-2cfd-42d1-996b-71424db6723e

3. Landi, Heather. "Amazon Care is shutting down at the end of 2022. Here's why." Fierce Healthcare. August 24, 2022. https://www.fiercehealthcare.com/health-tech/amazon-care-shutting-down-end-2022-tech-giant-said-virtual-primary-care-business-wasnt

4. Rosellini, Dr. Beth. "The Chiropractor-Dentist Collaboration: How we can help heal more patients in a way no one else can." Central Dentist. November 19, 2019. https://www.centraldentist.com/post/the-chiropractor-dentist-collaboration-how-we-can-help-heal-more-patients-in-a-way-no-one-else-can

5. Thielking, Megan. "Doctors are biased against patients. Is that a problem?" Stat. January 13, 2016. https://www.statnews.com/2016/01/13/doctors-bias/

6. "Biases in healthcare: An overview." Medical News Today. August 30, 2021. https://www.medicalnewstoday.com/articles/biases-in-healthcare

7. "Our Holistic Philosphy." Central Dentist. https://www.centraldentist.com/our-philosophy

8. Oberbrunner, Kary. Unhackable: The Elixir for Creating Flawless Ideas, Leveraging Superhuman Focus, and Achieving Optimal Human Performance. Ethos Collective. 2020.

9. Williams, Dr. Brownie. "Allergies and Behavior Problems in Children." Central Dentist. April 3, 2013. https://www.centraldentist.com/post/allergies-and-behavior-problems-in-children

10. Price, Weston A. *Nutrition and Physical Degeneration*. Price-Pottenger Nutrition Foundation, 2009.

HOLISTIC FAMILY DENTISTRY

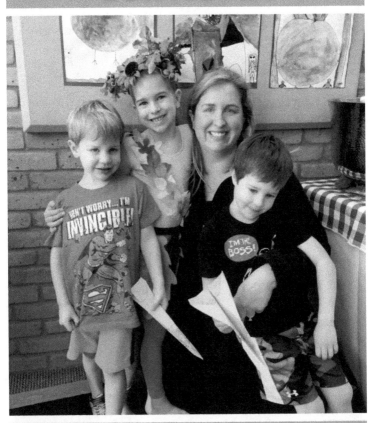

FIND OUT MORE AT:
CENTRALDENTIST.COM

INTERESTED IN FINDING OUT MORE ABOUT THE LATEST, MOST ADVANCED DENTAL TREATMENTS?

KEYNOTE SPEAKER

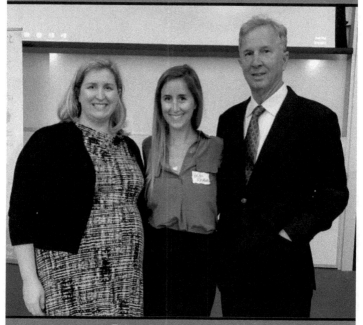

START THE CONVERSATION TODAY
CENTRALDENTIST.COM

CONNECT WITH JILL

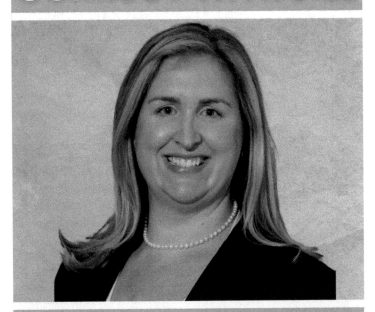

Follow her on your favorite
social media platforms today.

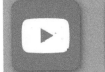 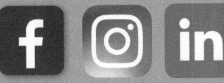

CENTRALDENTIST.COM

THIS BOOK IS PROTECTED INTELLECTUAL PROPERTY

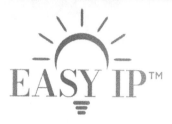

The author of this book values Intellectual Property. The book you just read is protected by Easy IP™, a proprietary process, which integrates blockchain technology giving Intellectual Property "Global Protection." By creating a "Time-Stamped" smart contract that can never be tampered with or changed, we establish "First Use" that tracks back to the author.

Easy IP™ functions much like a Pre-Patent™ since it provides an immutable "First Use" of the Intellectual Property. This is achieved through our proprietary process of leveraging blockchain technology and smart contracts. As a result, proving "First Use" is simple through a global and verifiable smart contract. By protecting intellectual property with blockchain technology and smart contracts, we establish a "First to File" event.

Powered By Easy IP™

LEARN MORE AT EASYIP.TODAY

Printed in the USA
CPSIA information can be obtained
at www.ICGtesting.com
LVHW080828070923
757252LV00003B/104